The Wellness Mindset:
5 Keys to Building Super Health

THE WELLNESS MINDSET

5 Keys to Building Super Health

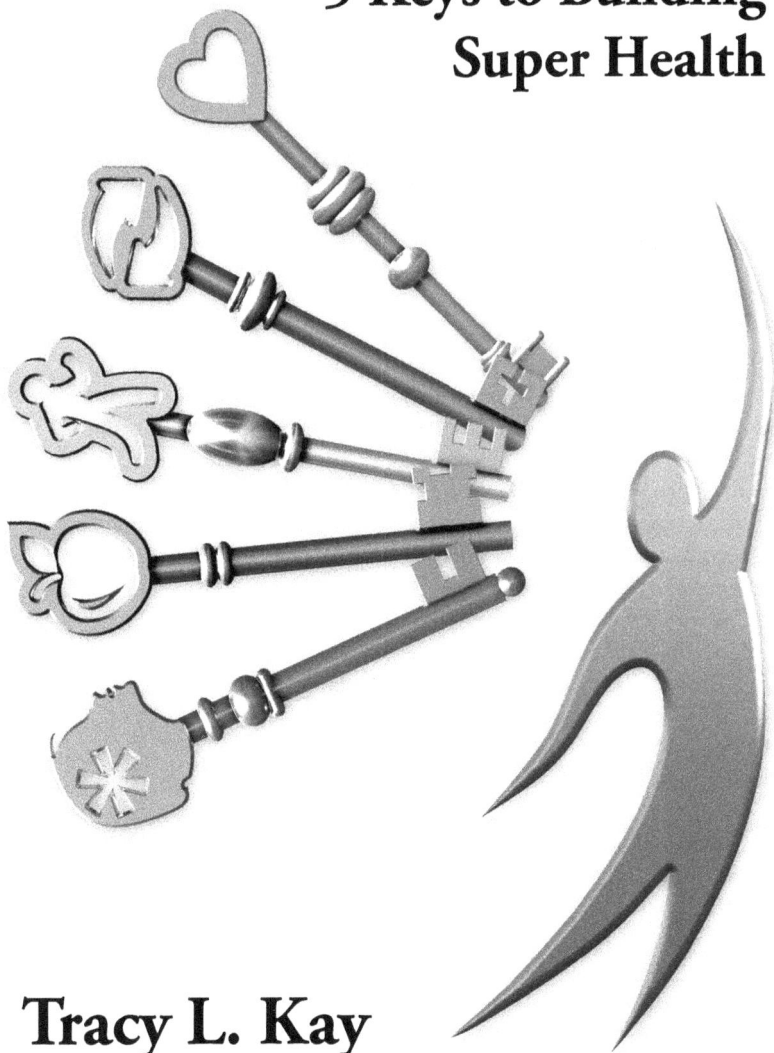

Tracy L. Kay

The Wellness Mindset: 5 Keys to Building Super Health

Cover artwork by Charlie Alolkoy
Editing and layout by Kira Freed

Kayholistics Publishing
21409 Falling Rock Terrace
Broadlands, VA 20148

ISBN: 978-0692357330

Printed in the United States of America

For Jeffrey,
who has been my rock
through the light and the darkness

"Let food be your medicine
and medicine be your food."

—Hippocrates

TABLE OF CONTENTS

INTRODUCTION

You don't have to be sick. That's right—you do not have to accept that as your body grows older, it will fall apart. It is possible to enjoy vibrant health for your entire life and have the energy to do anything your heart desires. If you have health challenges, it is possible to turn things around. It is possible to overcome these health challenges, even serious ones. Perhaps you've been told that you have to live with whatever is ailing you and that there's no hope of improvement. I'm here to tell you that you do not have to just live with it. Your body wants to be healthy, and it has an amazing capacity to heal if given the right tools. There is hope. I am living proof. You see, I was once told one of the scariest things in the world: "You have cancer." When you get news like that, it's as if the world stops. Then you ask yourself, "What do I do now?" Well, you can either fight or give up. I chose to fight for my health, and through this process I learned that it takes having the right mindset—the wellness mindset—and that there are keys you need to know about to walk in vibrant health. I vowed that once I emerged from the fire of ill health, I was going to help others do the same. If you are in this situation or are even just looking to improve your overall health, I wrote this book for you.

"The most delightful surprise
in life is to suddenly recognise
your own worth."
— Maxwell Maltz

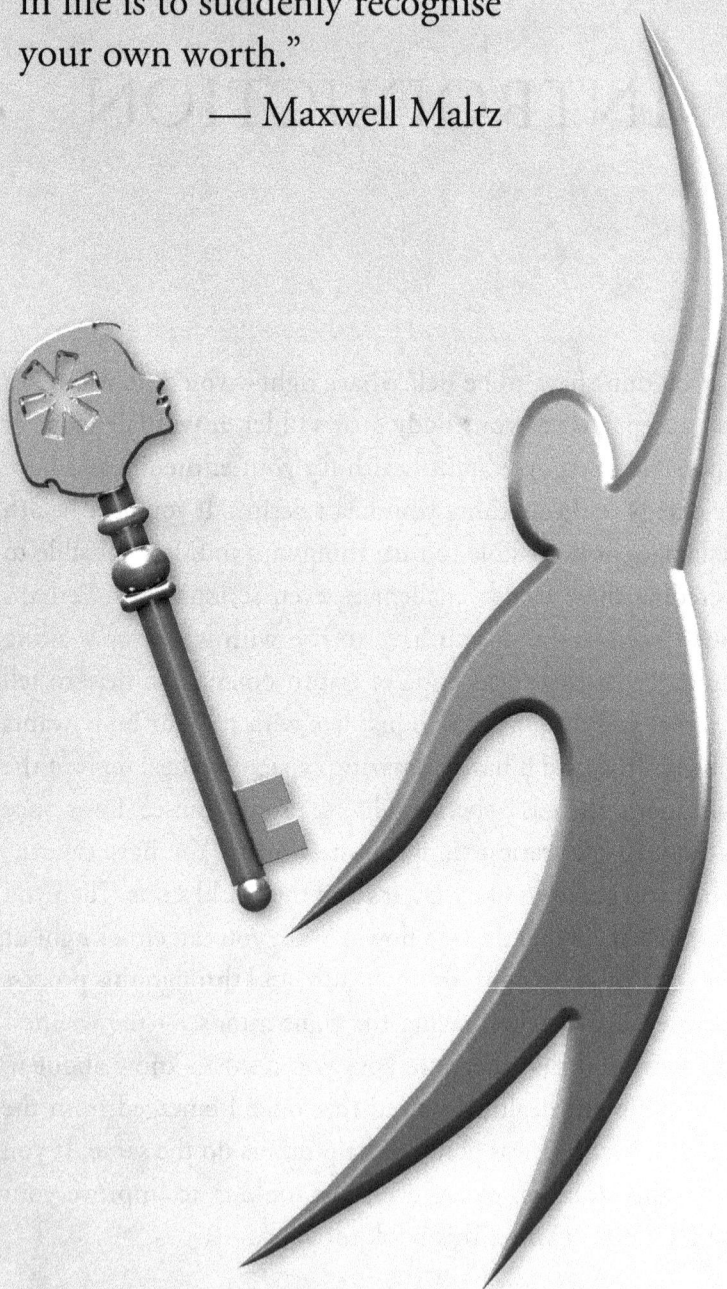

Key #1
VALUE YOURSELF

You have value. You have to believe that and internalize it. You are the only "you" in the world. Unique. Priceless. Never to be seen again. Knowing and accepting this fact should inform every choice that you make about your life. Once you understand that you have value, you will want to treat your body the best way possible. You will be more likely to make choices that enhance your health and well-being. You'll also likely spend your time doing things that enrich your life. You must accept this fact about yourself before you can fully achieve the vibrant, healthy body that you were meant to have. It all starts here.

Every day, say to yourself, "I have value." One technique you can use is to pay yourself a compliment. You simply say your name and then the compliment. For example, "Tracy, you have value, and there is no one else like you in the world!" or "Tracy, you are tenacious and will let nothing keep you from achieving your goals." The very act of doing this makes your subconscious mind think you are receiving a compliment from someone else. Your body then responds to that compliment in a positive way, just as if someone else actually did pay you a compliment. You see, your brain cannot differentiate between you paying yourself a compliment versus someone else. You can use this technique with any belief that you are looking to reinforce in yourself. It is invaluable for building your health. I do this every day, and I find that the best time to do it is just before drifting off to sleep at night. Doing this gives your subconscious mind the nighttime hours to internalize whatever you are focused on. My thanks to Dr. Henele E'ale of Genesis Energetic Health for sharing this technique with me.

When you understand that you have value, you begin to realize that your health is largely up to you. Take charge of your health! Make the commitment to yourself that you alone are responsible for your health. After all, you make the decision each day what to eat, whether to exercise and get the sleep you need, and all the rest. No one but you. You know, people will spend many thousands of dollars for a car and keep it in tiptop shape, but many will not consider spending a fraction of that amount to enhance their health. The car is replaceable, but your body is not! You must begin to see yourself as a worthy investment. It should be the first thing you invest in! No matter how much stuff you own, you cannot enjoy it if you are not in good health. In fact, your entire life is negatively impacted if you do not have your health. Don't let this happen to you. You want to be free to enjoy your life, and in order to do that to the fullest, you need to be in optimal health.

Become your own health advocate

Gather a team of medical professionals who practice different modalities. Many people tend to have one doctor they go to, and there is nothing wrong with that. But it's good not to put all your eggs in one basket. Instead, have more than one medical advisor, especially if you have a major health issue. When I was diagnosed with cancer, it was immensely helpful to have a team of medical professionals whom I trusted and could consult when deciding how to proceed. You really want to get your team in place, whether or not you have health issues and preferably before you do! You want your team to be diverse in the treatment approaches they deploy. Learn to take a balanced approach and open your mind to both conventional and complementary approaches. For instance, I have MDs, an ND (Naturopathic Doctor), and a Doctor of Oriental Medicine. These three types of practitioners provide different therapies for my health. Having these different points of view will help you make the best decisions for your health as well as become aware of things that can benefit you. If you only have one point of view, you limit yourself and can actually do yourself a disservice.

Really effective medical professionals, in my experience, tend to have certain traits in common:

◆ They are open minded and interested in the best approach to caring for your health, whether or not they recommended it.

◆ They are conversant in both conventional and alternative treatment methods.

◆ They actively listen to you and respect your viewpoint.

◆ They are quick to recommend lifestyle changes before prescribing drugs.

Become a lifelong student of health

Get in the habit of learning about health. Learn all you can. Read books and consider taking classes. In doing so, you will most likely discover an area of focus that you particularly enjoy and that helps you improve your health at the same time. In my case, I discovered that I had a knack for creating recipes for nutrient-dense dishes that are also delicious. As a result, I decided to increase my knowledge in this area. Today, I am a graduate of the Matthew Kenney Academy, where I studied culinary nutrition. Best of all, I was able to do it online. I have included some great reference materials on this and other resources I use at the back of this book to help you get started. They have served me well, and I believe they will also be helpful to you.

"Don't eat anything your great-grandmother wouldn't recognize as food."

— Michael Pollan

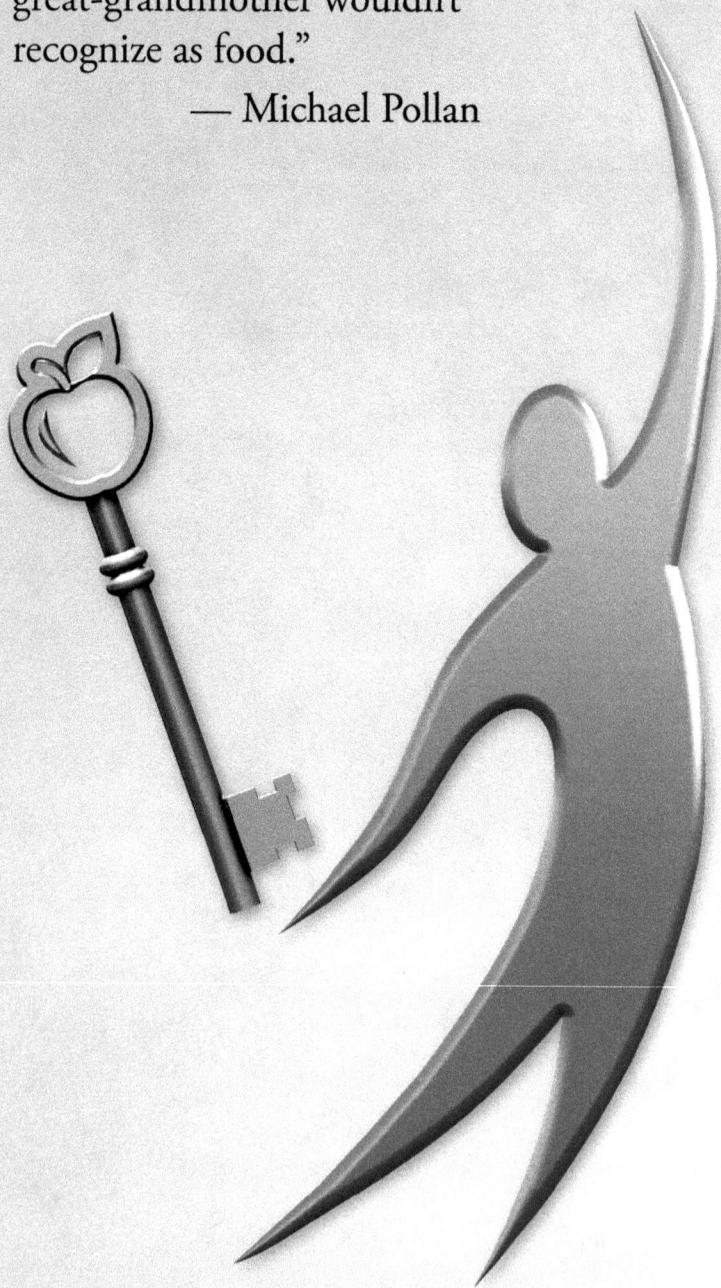

Key #2

EAT AS IF YOUR LIFE
DEPENDS ON IT!

The food you consume is the cornerstone of building super health in your body. When it comes to food, there is no middle ground. It's black or it's white—there's no gray area. The food you eat either builds health or it doesn't. That is the stance you have to take with everything you eat, especially if you have a serious health challenge, as I did.

Invest in the best food you can afford

Purchase organic fruits and vegetables that are locally grown, if possible. If you eat meat and fish, look for grass-fed beef and wild-caught fish. I realize that it's not always possible to purchase exclusively organic, but do your best and keep in mind that the quality of what you put into your body matters! You can have the ultimate in organic, locally grown produce if you garden at home. Even if you don't have much room, you can still grow a substantial amount of food at home. For instance, I grow much of my produce right on my deck using a minimum of space. I have included information on how I do that in the Resources section at the back of this book. Growing food at home also gives you the advantage of having truly vine-ripened food. Why is this important? Well, did you know that many of the phytonutrients in fruits and vegetables are developed in the last 20 percent of the time they spend on the vine? When you buy produce from the grocery store, it is not vine ripened because it must travel great distances, in most cases, before it reaches you. It must be harvested before it ripens or else it would rot by the time it reached the grocery store. This is also true for all commercially produced produce, whether conventionally grown or organic. As a result, many of the fruits and vegetables that you purchase can be lacking in many phytonutrients. That, coupled with the fact that much of the soil that food is grown in today is nutrient deficient, makes it all the more important to consider home gardening. With that said, if you purchase produce from a grocery store, organic is still the better choice because it will be more nutrient rich and freer of contaminants than standard commercially grown produce.

You do indeed become what you eat because your body uses what you consume to repair your cells, provide you with energy, and build your immune system, among many other functions. The old saying "Garbage in, garbage out" or GIGO, is very true here. Eat junk, become junk. But that won't be you because you value yourself! Begin to be really picky about what you put into your body. Remember, your health depends on it.

Planning your daily sustenance ranks right up there with breathing. If you fail to plan, you will fail—that's just the way it goes. Running out the door in the morning and grabbing something just won't cut it. You need to start your day with nutrient-dense food. One of the best ways I've found to do that is to make a smoothie. Smoothies are great because you can pack a huge amount of nutrients in a fairly small package.

And because they are blended, the food is broken down into a more easily usable form so the body can better absorb the nutrients. Flavor combinations are endless, but a basic smoothie will consist of a base liquid like dairy or nut milk or juice, fruits, and berries. For extra nutritional power, I like to do what I call "tank it up." This involves adding extra ingredients to boost the smoothie's nutrient content. I add things like greens—for example, spinach or kale—and superfoods like turmeric. Turmeric is a plant that originated in Southeast Asia and contains a substance called curcumin, which offers numerous health benefits, including being an anti-inflammatory. I buy it fresh from the produce department at my local Whole Foods.

Superfoods are unparalleled for adding incredible nutrition to a smoothie or a meal. They are called "super" because they have an extraordinarily high nutrients-to-serving ratio and because a very small amount goes a long way. So, it is not necessary to add a large quantity of these to be effective. After all, the body can only absorb just so much at once. There are many superfoods, and an exhaustive list is beyond the scope of this book. However, here are the ones I use most often:

- ◆ **Maca** is a plant native to the Andes. It comes as a powder and is rich in amino acids, vitamins, minerals, fatty acids, and proteins. It has sort of a butterscotch flavor.

- ◆ **Cacao nibs** are crumbled raw cacao beans. They provide the rich taste of chocolate and are loaded with antioxidants, vitamins, minerals, and fiber. In addition to putting them in smoothies, I add them to my morning steel-cut oats cereal. Yum!

- **Lucuma** is a sweet fruit from the lucuma tree that contains beta-carotene, zinc, niacin, and iron. It comes in powder form and has a banana-like flavor.

- **Goji berries** are one of the most antioxidant-rich foods on the planet. They are small, chewy red berries that add a great flavor to a smoothie. Since the flavor of these berries is both sweet and savory, they can also be added to a wide variety of dishes. I even put them in my vegan chile!

- **Hemp seeds** are one of the oldest foods in the world. They contain all the essential amino acids, which makes them a vegan source of complete protein. In addition, they are loaded with omega-3 and omega-6 fatty acids.

- **Chia seeds** are tiny seeds that have a slightly nutty flavor. They are loaded with protein and fiber as well as being a great source of omega-3 and omega-6 fats. They can absorb up to 10 times their weight in liquid and add a nice thickness to smoothies. The ancient Maya would eat chia seeds before going into battle.

- **Flaxseeds** are fantastic for adding omega-3 fats and fiber to your diet. Not only are they great in smoothies, but they are also a great addition to baked goods like muffins.

On the next page is the recipe for my daily smoothie. I will add other ingredients as the mood strikes me, but this is the basic recipe. Feel free to be creative and make it your own. Just be sure to include both berries and greens in your smoothie. These foods pack a powerful nutritional punch. Berries, in particular, are loaded with antioxidants that are very protective for your health, and greens are an excellent source of nutrients like vitamins A, C, K, and folate as well as minerals like potassium and calcium. I feel amazing after I have one of these smoothies! Now, it won't look pretty, but you are in it for the nutrition, not how it looks.

Tracy's Tanked-Up Smoothie

½ medium banana

1 cup frozen blueberries or any other berry that you like (or use a combination!)

1 cup almond milk or any unsweetened non-dairy milk of your choice

1 tsp. maca

1 thumb-sized piece of turmeric

1 cup fresh spinach or other greens

1 tbsp. chia, hemp, or flaxseeds

½ tsp. vanilla

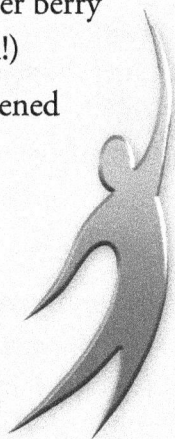

I encourage you to invest in a really good blender. My recommendation is either Vitamix or Blendtec. I have used both, and they are fantastic for quickly breaking down and liquefying the smoothie ingredients. This is important because it makes it easier for the body to absorb the nutrients, particularly something like kale, which requires breaking down the cell wall in order get the maximum nutrition. If those machines are not in your budget, I also like and have used the Nutri-Bullet. It does a fairly good job of liquefying ingredients; however, it will take longer.

The same planning you do for breakfast also needs to be done for lunch and dinner. Don't go out to the local "choke and puke" and throw down a sandwich made of who knows what! What you want to do is to plan your meals so that they are nutrient dense. For instance, for lunch, consider a salad with vegetables of all the colors of the rainbow. The more color in your salad, the more nutrients you'll get. If you don't like salads, I encourage you to learn to like them because they are a great way to get large amounts of phytonutrients into your body.

Eat phytonutrient-rich meals

Phytonutrients are the key for both prevention and reversal of diseases like heart disease and diabetes.

Your immune system's job is to protect you, and phytonutrients play a vital role in keeping it strong. Another great benefit is that getting enough of these nutrients turns off what I like to call the "hunger monster." Most of us have met him, I believe. He's the one that lives in your stomach and growls that he is still hungry after you've eaten so that you continue to eat more than your body needs. This is mainly what sabotages any attempt to take off excess weight. Phytonutrients shut down the hunger monster because your body is getting what it needs, so it no longer needs to growl, as it were, for more food. Your appetite will begin to normalize. Try it and see if I'm not right. I know it worked for me because I took off nearly 50 pounds without being hungry at any time. I couldn't believe how simple it was. It was just from food, not gimmicks. Oh, and I ate as much as I wanted. Is that great or what?

As much as I enjoy salads, I cannot subsist on those alone. So, one of the many tools that I use for meal planning is the cookbook *Eat to Live* by Dr. Joel Fuhrman. It provides many options for healthy breakfasts, lunches, and dinners as well as guidelines for creating phytonutrient-rich meals. Please note that whether or not you eat animal proteins, fruits and vegetables are the only foods that contain these vital nutrients. You might be thinking, "But I take vitamin supplements!" Well, did you know that vitamin supplements really do not do anything to protect you from chronic diseases? Several studies have shown that taking vitamin and mineral supplements has no effect on preventing strokes, heart disease, or other ailments like cancer. In some cases, they can even cause harm. When you consider that consumers invest over $30 billion a year in the supplement industry, that's a mountain of pills, and many people are buying them under the mistaken impression that these products will safeguard their health. I know—I was one of them. I must have spent hundreds if not thousands of dollars on supplements over the years, and I still got cancer! This may come as a real bummer to many of you reading this, but there is good news! If you strive get these nutrients from your food, you can and will build your health in such a way as to put yourself in the best position to prevent disease.

Be aware that sometimes supplementation could be indicated, depending on your circumstances, because each of us is unique. I work with my medical professionals to ensure that I avoid deficiencies, and I recommend that you do the same. Remember, though, fruits and vegetables are the very best sources of these nutrients. If you strive to eat phytonutrient-rich meals, you should need very little supplementation. So, how much do you need to consume daily? The current recommendation by the U.S. Department of Agriculture (USDA) says 7–13 servings a day. A serving is about half a cup, and if you have any health challenges, you want to be on the higher end of that range. I strive to eat that many servings a day, and I also take a food-based fruit, vegetable, and berry nutritional product daily. I do this because given the stressful, hectic lives we live today, in my opinion, you cannot get enough of these vital nutrients if you want to safeguard your health. I have included information on this in the Resources section at the back of this book.

Also, in the very act of just living, you undergo something called oxidative stress. Simply put, this is the damage that your cells—essentially, your DNA—are subjected to every day of your life. This damage is the precursor to disease. A practical example of this is what happens when you cut into an apple. At first, the cut surfaces are perfectly white, but wait a few minutes and you'll notice that they begin to turn brown. That's oxidation. Now, what happens if, after you slice the apple, you sprinkle on some fresh lemon juice? You'll notice that the apple does not turn brown. Why? The lemon juice contains antioxidant phytochemicals that protect against oxidation. In much the same way, when you consume plenty of phytonutrients from fruits and vegetables, they protect you against oxidation and even assist your body in repairing much of this type of damage.

"Those who think they have no time for exercise will sooner or later have to find time for illness."
— Edward Stanley

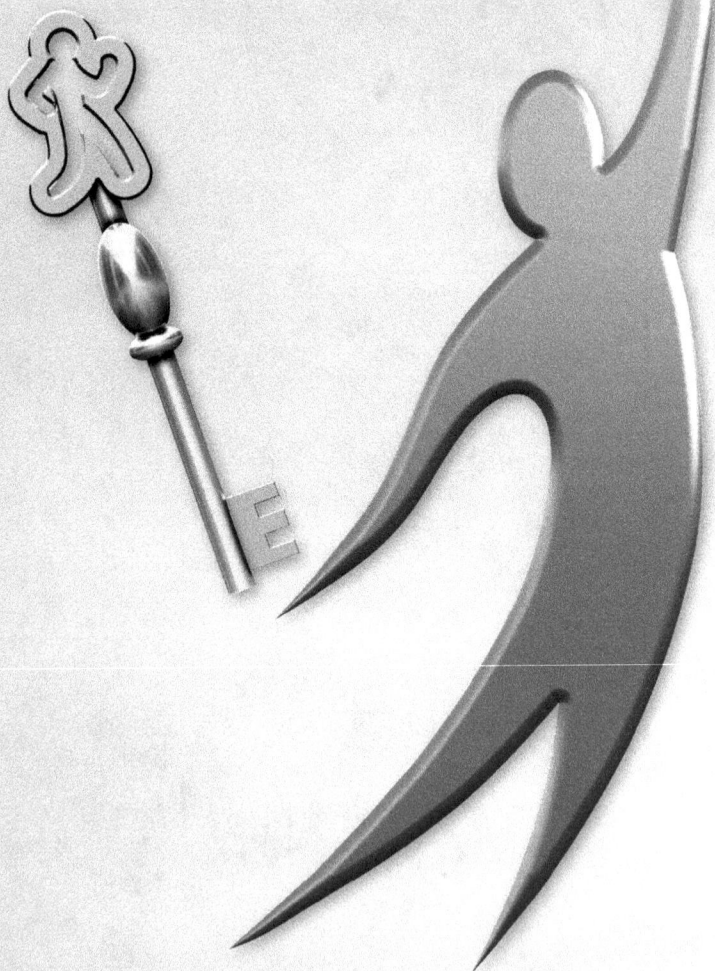

Key #3
MOVE IT!

As a song by the legendary James Brown says, "Get up off of that thing and move and you'll feel better"! Well, I did paraphrase a bit. This is hugely important. You must move every day. Get started with something. Walking is a great place to start. If you can only do 10 steps today, then do 11 tomorrow. Keep building until you are walking far. If walking is not your thing, find something you else you like, but do something! You also want to think about varying the types of exercises that you do. For instance, I have found it helpful to do cardio, yoga, and some strength training. It's not good to do the same thing all the time because the body gets accustomed to it. For example, cardio will benefit your heart but will not do anything for flexibility, as yoga would. Exercise strengthens your immune system and is imperative for healthy elimination. Not to be indelicate here, but, well, pooping is all-important, as your body rids itself of a great many toxins this way. So you want to keep things moving, if you know what I mean. Moving also floods your body with oxygen. It will also help you to sleep better and have more energy. Please be sure, though, to check with your medical professionals before commencing any exercise program, especially if you have any physical challenges.

Don't sit all day

Sitting and being sedentary are the enemies of super health. If you do either to excess, you will most likely set yourself up for potential health problems. Did you know that sitting for many hours a day is the equivalent of cigarette smoking? In fact, there is a growing body of research showing that the amount of sitting you do has a direct impact on your health.

If you sit at a desk all day, get up and move at least once per hour. If you have somewhere you can walk, that's great. If not, at least get up and stretch and stay standing for at least 15 minutes before sitting down again. I remember the strange looks I would get when I would speed walk around the indoor atrium in my former office building. But, hey, I started a trend. Soon I noticed others walking as well.

If you do not have the option to stay standing for 15 minutes, consider exercises that can be done at your desk while sitting. Believe it or not, there are many great exercises that can be done while sitting at a desk. One of the things I like to do is lift one leg at a time and do ankle rotations. This really helps the circulation in the legs. I also try to stretch both arms overhead at least five times per hour. I find that this relieves tension in my neck and shoulders. A great way to find inspiration to get started is to Google "desk exercises."

A final word about exercise: please do not neglect to nourish your body with plenty of phytonutrients. Yes, exercise is very important, but it will not make up for a poor diet. The late, great Jack LaLanne once famously said, "Exercise is king. Nutrition is queen. Put them together and you've got a kingdom."

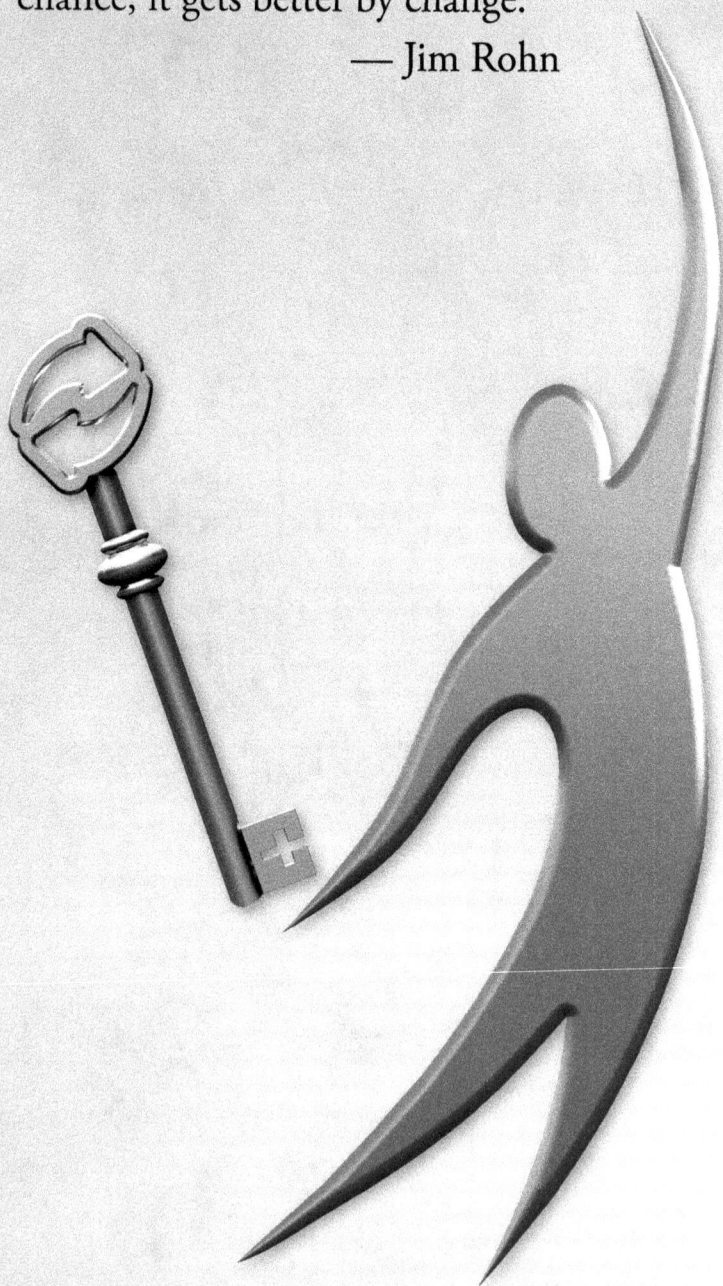

"Your life does not get better by
chance, it gets better by change."
— Jim Rohn

Key #4
MAKE A CHANGE!

I 've already talked about what you eat and the importance of moving every day. Now we have to talk about your life in general. If you want your health to be different, you must be different. Everything you do, say, think, and eat must change. There is a famous quotation that I think is so appropriate here: "If you want what you do not have in your life, you must do what you have never done." In other words, you must reinvent yourself. In June of 2013, when I was diagnosed with cancer, I was significantly overweight. I had horrible back pain, and I was on some serious pain medication around the clock. I was always tired and stressed. After hearing the news that I had cancer, I resolved to do everything in my power to regain my health. I learned that I had to become a new "me," so I did. Here are the main things to know:

Learn gratitude

When was the last time you were truly thankful for the blessings in your life? We all get so busy, and many times we fail to see that we are truly blessed in many ways. I want to encourage you to learn gratitude. Be thankful for every day that you have. Take some time each day to reflect on the good things in your life. Doing this will put you in a positive frame of mind each time you do it. Do your best to avoid negative thoughts. Remember, where the mind goes, the body follows! What do I mean by that? Well, let me ask you this: have you ever noticed that when you are in a negative frame of mind, you start feeling tired, or conversely, when you are in a positive state of mind, you generally feel pretty good? Your state of mind can indeed greatly affect how you feel physically. Now, I know what's it like to feel ill physically, but I quickly learned that a negative mindset was not going to help me feel any better, so I resolved to keep my thoughts as positive as I possibly could. Looking for things to be thankful for definitely helps.

Get rid of toxic situations and people in your life

You know, those people who are always negative about everything. They may even put you down or criticize everything you do. These are people who will generally be hypercritical of any effort you make to improve your health, especially if they do not agree with the path you choose to take to accomplish this. Sadly, they may even be close family members. No matter who they are, start giving them a wide berth. Try to spend as little time as you can around them. Doing this doesn't mean that you don't love them, but you have to take no prisoners where your health is concerned, especially if you are facing a serious health challenge.

You have one life—make it work for you

If you are in a job or relationship or any other situation that causes you stress, over time that can negatively affect your health as well. Reducing the stress in your life is something you should deal with immediately. I know from experience that this is not easy to do, but you should consider making changes if you are unhappy. Remember, you only have one life, and it's not worth it to be miserable. Here are the steps to follow to make the needed changes:

◆ First, begin to think about what you want in a job, relationship, or any other area of your life that doesn't feel satisfying.

◆ Second, write these things down. Be very specific.

◆ Third, look at what you wrote every day and think about it in order to keep it on your mind.

Have you ever noticed that when you concentrate or focus on something, somehow it comes to pass? This is a simplistic example, but has it ever happened to you that you thought about wanting a particular item and then suddenly you start noticing this item everywhere you go—it seems as though it is everywhere! Then an opportunity pops up for you to obtain it. It can seem like magic, but it's not. It's just that your eyes are now open to whatever it is you are concentrating on and the opportunities to get whatever it is you are after.

"Did you know that putting chemicals on your skin can be far worse than ingesting them?"
— Dr. Joseph Mercola

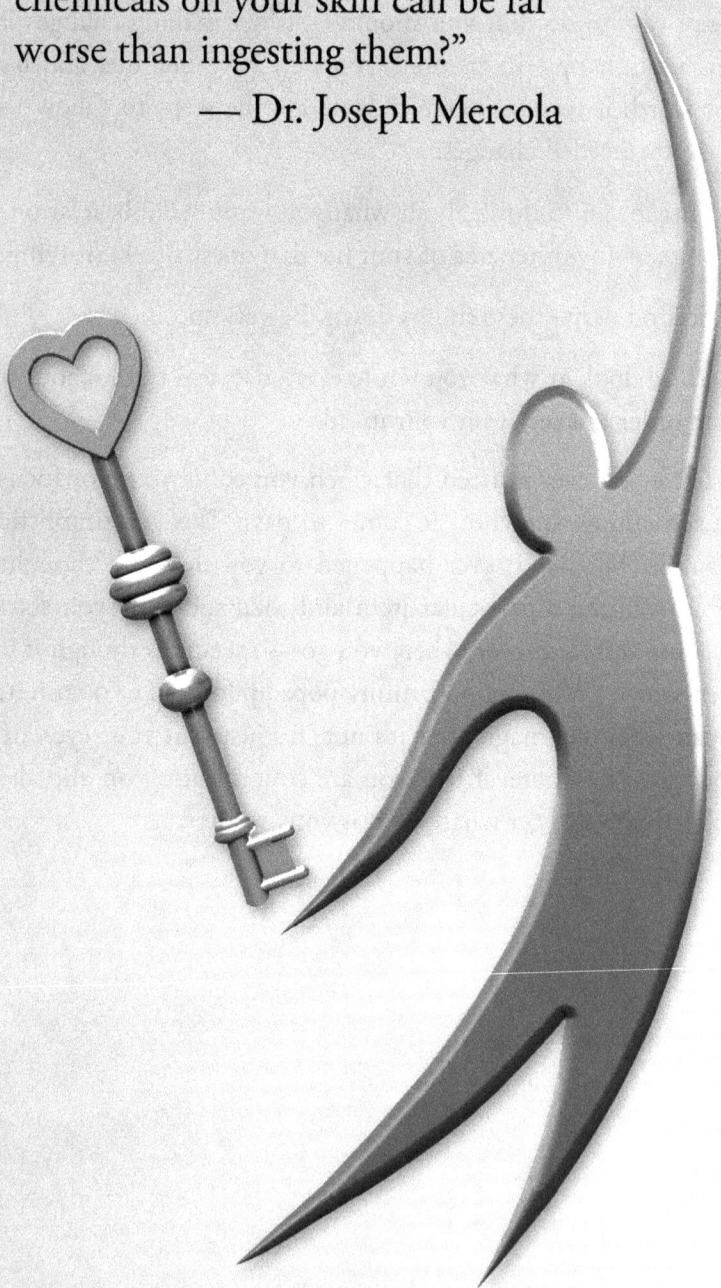

Key #5

SELF-CARE

When was the last time you gave serious consideration to the daily care you give your body? By that, I mean everything from the personal care products you use to your nightly rest. Many times we spend our days rushing around with little thought to the care of the miraculous machine that enables us to do all we do. Part of super health is taking time every day to give your body some TLC. Here are some important things to consider.

Body care

Taking care of yourself includes giving careful consideration to the personal care products you use. I used to believe that the products I used must be safe or else they wouldn't be for sale to the general public. I have since found out that this is not always true. Every day I would bathe and perfume myself in my scent of the moment and then proceed to use every face potion known to man and then put on my war paint (that's code for makeup). I was and still am a cosmetics junkie and, back in the day, gave little thought to the impact these products could be having on my health. If it smelled good, looked good, and I thought it would make me look fabulous, I had to have it! These days, I still indulge the junkie in me, but I am very choosy as to what products I purchase and use. This is an area you really need to pay attention to if you are serious about safeguarding your health. And you are, right? After all, you have value, and nothing less will do.

Do you know what is in the products you use on your body? I'm talking about the personal care products that you apply to your body when you get ready for your day. Why is this important? Because your skin will absorb at least 80 percent of what you put on it. If the products you use contain ingredients that you can't pronounce or would not eat, consider not putting them on your skin—especially if you are facing a serious illness. Many of the chemicals in skin care products are, in fact, toxic. One of the most dangerous is fragrance. Did you know that when you see the word *fragrance* on a label that the product in question could contain dozens or more of these chemicals that the manufacturer is not required by the Food and Drug Administration (FDA) to list on the label? Yet many of these chemicals are highly toxic. The more of these chemicals you use, the more your immune system has to marshal its defenses to protect you from them. Your immune system is your defense when fighting any illness. You do not want to tax it needlessly with harmful chemicals. For this reason, consider eliminating products that contain fragrance and other potentially toxic ingredients, including:

- ◆ **Bronopol, DMDM hydantoin, diazolidinyl urea, imidazolidinyl urea, and quaternium-15:** All of these compounds are what is known as formaldehyde releasers. Not only is formaldehyde a known carcinogenic to humans, but it can also trigger allergic skin reactions. These ingredients are found in many personal products.

Commonly found in: shampoos, conditioners, lotions, cosmetics.

◆ **Parabens:** These substances may disrupt the endocrine system and contribute to reproductive and developmental problems. Parabens are used extensively in the personal care world mostly because they are relatively inexpensive preservatives, so you will need to be really vigilant when reading labels.

Commonly found in: cosmetics, antiperspirants, moisturizers, shampoos, conditioners.

◆ **Phthalates:** One of the things that phthalates are used for is to add flexibility and resistance to chipping in nail polish. There is evidence showing that these chemicals can damage the reproductive system, and phthalates can "hide" behind fragrance in products. This is yet another reason to avoid fragrance.

Commonly found in: nail polish, perfume, deodorant, hair spray.

◆ **BHA and BHT:** Avoid these like the plague, as they are suspected human carcinogens. These are found in a wide variety of products and can be used as preservatives in food. Yummy! Not.

Commonly found in: Cosmetics, hair products, sunscreen, fragrance, creams, antiperspirants, deodorant.

◆ **Toluene:** This is used as a solvent and is commonly used in nail polish. It has been linked to toxicity to the immune system—something you definitely don't want when working to build your health!

◆ **Methylisothiazolinone, methylchloroisothiazolinone, and benzisothiazolinone:** These substances are commonly used in shampoos, soaps, hand creams, and moisturizers. They are preservatives that can cause contact allergies and may be neurotoxic. Stay, far, far, away!

◆ **Sulfates (sodium lauryl sulfate, sodium laureth sulfate):** These are used as foaming agents in shampoos, toothpastes, and soaps, and can cause skin and eye irritation. There is also an indication that sulfates can damage the immune system, as shown by a study reported in the *International Journal of Toxicology*, which is published by the American College of Toxicology. Again, give a wide berth to anything that can compromise your immune system.

Pretty scary stuff, huh? And it get even better. No one knows the cumulative effects of using these chemicals in combination over time because how do you even begin to test this when people use multiple products daily with a myriad of ingredients? This is tantamount to chemical warfare being waged against your body every day! So what should you use? Look for products that contain few ingredients. Again, if you would not eat it, do not put it on your skin. If you are ill, remember that you want to keep your immune system as unburdened as possible. You need it to be strong. There are safe products out there. An excellent resource to use to check what substances are in the products you use is www.ewg.org, the website of the Environmental Working Group. They have a cosmetics database that contains a wide variety of products by hundreds of manufacturers and also provide tips on what to avoid in personal care products. I am also including some resources for safe products in the Resources section at the back of this book.

While considering what personal care products to use, you also want to take a look at the products you use to clean your home. Many of the toxic ingredients listed above are also in home care products. Look for products that are nontoxic because what you use in your home will also have an effect on your health. Check out EWG's healthy home tips at www.ewg. org/healthyhometips for recommendations on how to avoid toxic cleaning products and other tips on reducing toxicity in your home.

Sleep

Don't neglect it. Sleep is one of the most powerful tools that your body uses to repair and regenerate. Your body will not function at its best without adequate sleep. Benjamin Franklin famously said, "Early to bed and early to rise makes a man healthy, wealthy, and wise." I'm not sure about the wealthy part, but adequate sleep certainly is wise. Get yourself in bed no later than 10:30 p.m. The goal here is to be asleep long before midnight because midnight and later is when your body begins its repair work. You want to make sure that you are asleep during this time or else you will disrupt this important work. Put down that computer or book, and record that TV show to watch later. You need to get your sleep.

Now, if sleep is not coming easy to you, it's time to investigate the cause. For instance, how much coffee did you have today, and when did you have your last cup? Coffee contains the stimulant caffeine, and enough of that can certainly disrupt your sleep. How about sodas? They also can contain a significant amount of caffeine. What time was your last meal of the day? Eating too late can also keep you awake.

Another thing to consider that plagues many people is the inability to shut off your thoughts—you know, when thousands of thoughts are swirling through your head, and you can't shut them off, especially when you are worried about something? If, like me, you have experienced this, I've found it helpful to develop a nightly routine that helps prepare me for sleep. Now, you don't have to do what I do—everyone is different. But I've found that if I turn off all electronics at least one hour before bed and take a warm bath, it sets me up for a good night's sleep.

Something else I found helpful is thinking of things I'm thankful for. Remember gratitude from earlier? It works great before you go to bed because it puts you in a great frame of mind and helps you forget about your troubles, both of which are helpful in promoting a good night's sleep.

Another trick, which I learned from my grandmother, is to "fling" my problems to the floor before going to sleep. She would actually ball up her problems in her hands, as if they were physical objects, and toss them to the floor. She told me that oftentimes the solutions to her problems would come to her the next day when she woke up. I've tried this, and if my problems weren't solved the next day, I at least experienced a release from thinking about my troubles. The point is to come up with a routine that works for you.

What you sleep on and in are just as important. I use organic cotton or bamboo sheets and stay away from synthetic materials. Anything with synthetic materials will most likely contain toxic chemicals, and you don't want those anywhere near you, especially where you spend at least one-third of your life—in bed. My entire bed is even organic. Did you know that most mattresses contain harmful chemicals due to the fact that they are required by federal law to contain flame-retardant chemicals. You do not want these anywhere near you! Also, many mattresses are made with petrochemicals that outgas. Why would you want to be bombarded with toxic chemicals as you sleep?

Are you in the habit of sleeping with your cell phone by the bed? Consider moving it elsewhere, as the radiation coming from that phone is not good for you to be near. Move your phone to another room and charge it there. Keeping electronics away from you when you sleep is much healthier for you.

Take a bath

Here in America, we are shower mad! We are some of the cleanest people in the world. Now, showers are useful, of course, for keeping clean, but there is nothing like a nice bath. It can provide some real benefits. First, the very act of soaking in the tub is very relaxing, and relaxation, in my view, is something we could all use more of. Second, you can put beneficial things in the tub to help this process. One of the things I like to use is a lavender bath bomb. It adds to the relaxation of the bath and softens my skin. If you do this before bed, you should sleep well. I know I do!

Something else to do while you are in the bath is to exfoliate your skin. There are some really great nontoxic products out there to use for this purpose. (I include them in the Resources section.) Your skin is your body's largest eliminative organ, and exfoliating will get rid of dead skin and encourage new cells to turn over faster, which makes your skin look more youthful. Who wouldn't love that?

"The more serious the illness, the more important it is for you to fight back, mobilizing all your resources—spiritual, emotional, intellectual, physical."

— Norman Cousins

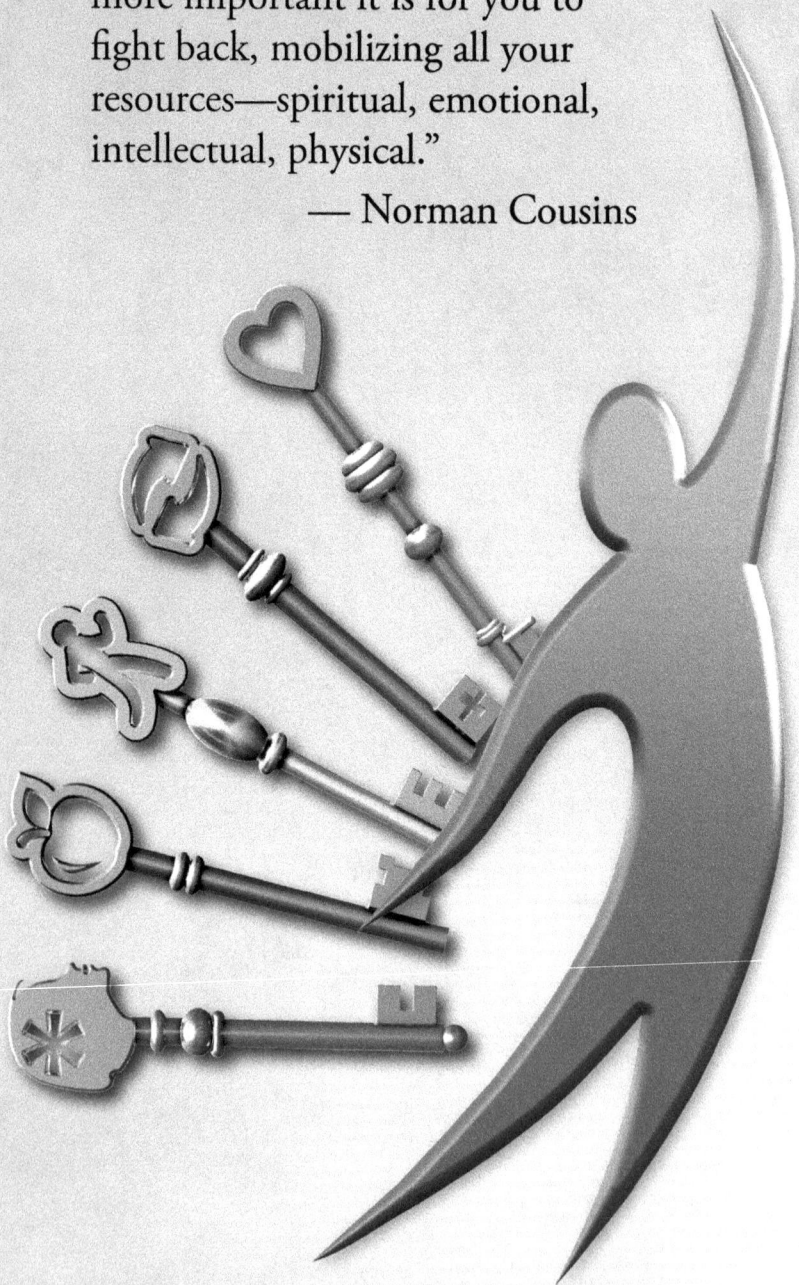

What to Do if You Are Diagnosed with a Serious Illness

I f you have been diagnosed with a serious illness, my heart goes out to you. The first thing you want to do is take a deep breath and try not to panic. Panicking can cause you to make hasty decisions, which could adversely affect your health in the long run. Taking time to gather information before making any decisions greatly improves your chances for success. So here are the two main things you want to do:

1. Get your medical team in place. If you have not done this, now is the time to get your medical advisors together. Depending on what you are facing, your team could consist of oncologists, cardiologists, or other specialists. You also want to ensure that, as I mentioned in Key #1, you have medical professionals who are open minded.

2. Develop a get-well plan and a stay-well plan.

The medical professionals you choose must be able help you with your get-well plan and stay-well plan. But please understand that your oncologist, cardiologist, or other specialists are interested in one thing, which is killing the disease in your body. They are not generally focused on treating your body as a whole—that is, supporting your body through whatever treatments you are undergoing. Their sole mission is to destroy whatever is threatening your health and life. It's not that they don't care about your general health; it's just that medical school doesn't tend to teach doctors much about alternative treatments and nutrition. This is where you have to become your own health advocate. You have to ensure that you are also supporting your immune system throughout your treatment. Remember, the treatment is ONLY designed to kill the disease. Your immune system is what fights for you and gets you well, and you must take every step to protect and strengthen it! This is where it is extremely important to obtain the advice of health-care professionals who are proficient in alternative therapies that can complement your treatment—hence, your get-well plan. Here is what you need to consider for your personal get-well plan:

- ◆ What conventional and/or alternative therapies will you use? Some people will tell you that you need to use only alternative therapies in your treatment, and others will tell you that you need to use only conventional methods. I have found, at least in my case, that it takes a combination of the two. Everyone is different, and you have to assess your own situation, but by and large this will most likely be the case. Remember, you want medical professionals who are open minded. For instance, I was fortunate to have oncologists who were open to whatever alternative treatments I wanted to use as long as those treatments didn't interfere with what they were doing for me. They were open minded and willing to let me incorporate treatments from my other health-care professionals, such as acupuncture and Chinese herbs. This goes back to what I said earlier in the book. I cannot stress enough the importance of supporting your body throughout your treatment. Always remember that you are the one who decides how to proceed. Your medical team makes recommendations, but you have the final say.

◆ Plan meals so you get plenty of phytonutrients. If you didn't eat as though your life depended on it before, hop to it now! You need phytonutrients by the barrelful to strengthen your immunity. No matter what conventional and/or alternative treatments you choose, do not neglect to feed your body these vital nutrients. And where do you get these? Fruits and vegetables, of course! This is where you want to adopt a whole-food diet, as I discussed earlier. This is no time to be playing Russian roulette with your diet and lifestyle. This is "all hands on deck" time. Take no prisoners. Planning is especially important here and, depending on the treatments you are undergoing, will determine how you get those phytonutrients into your diet. For instance, in my case, I had to avoid a lot of fiber during treatment. This is where the whole-food nutritional product I mentioned under Key #2 was so valuable. If eating solid food is difficult, consider incorporating smoothies and soups. I've already talked about smoothies, but soups are another excellent way to pack in an abundance of vital nutrients. They are also very soothing. It's better to make soups yourself, or if it's easier for you to buy prepackaged products, I have included some recommendations in the Resources section at the back of this book. It is simple, however, to make a quick, nourishing soup at home. It's as simple as combining a cup of low-sodium vegetable broth with a few fresh vegetables in a high-speed blender. Use a blender to make soup? You bet! I have used both the VitaMix and Blendtec machines to make soup. Just as when making smoothies, using a high-speed blender like either of these appliances breaks down the cell walls in the vegetables and makes it easier for your body to absorb the nutrients. You simply add your ingredients and let the blender run for 6–8 minutes, which warms the soup. Here is a simple recipe to get you started:

Simple Carotene-Rich Soup

1 cup organic low-sodium vegetable broth

1 medium carrot chopped

1/2 medium red bell pepper

1/4 celery root

1/2 medium tomato

1/2 cup spinach or kale

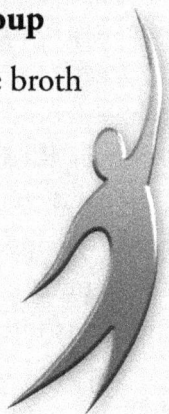

You also want to ensure that you get a large amount of greens in your diet. Now, if eating these is not your favorite, you are not alone. Some good tricks for getting this vital food into your diet include blending them into soups (as in the recipe above) and smoothies as well as eating kale chips. If you've never tried them, they are quite addicting. They can be found in health food stores and many mainstream grocery stores, and they come in many flavors. You want to be sure to look for those that have been dehydrated at low temperatures so as to preserve the nutrients. I have included my recommendation in the Resources section.

◆ **Get adequate sleep and stay positive.** Most of us need at least eight hours of sleep, and you may need more. If you need a nap, take it. It is important to listen to your body and rest when you are tired. Get the sleep you need in order to keep your mind in a good place, and stay away from toxic people and situations. This is especially crucial when you are working to regain your health. Remember, where the mind goes, the body follows. You can have days when you feel low physically and sometimes also mentally, and that's okay—it happens. We are human, after all. The thing to remember here is that when you are feeling negative, recognize it and deal with it. Are you feeling afraid, angry, or just plain frustrated? Maybe you are experiencing all those emotions at once. I know I did, and even though I was blessed to be surrounded by all of the love and support I could ever hope for, I still felt as though I was alone at times. When negative thoughts like these would begin to crowd my thinking, I would stop and immediately think of the things I could be thankful for—things like thanking God for blessing me with good doctors, loved ones who were there for me, and so on. That alone will help lift you out of the doldrums.

◆ **Exercise.** Next, get up and move as you are able to. In my case, it helped me to take a short walk outside and go as far as I could, even when it was raining! Some days were better than others. The key thing to keep in mind is that while there are times when you may feel really bad, those times will not last. You will have better times and days.

◆ ◆ ◆

Now let's fast-forward, and let's say you got the good news that you are now disease-free. Congratulations! You have been through a lot to get to this point. Now what do you do? You may think, "I get to rest now. I worked so hard to get better that I can take a break and celebrate with whatever food and party hearty and do basically whatever I want." You could not be more wrong! Now is not the time to let down your guard. Nope. Now it's time to implement your stay-well plan.

The stay-well plan is essentially the get-well plan minus the treatments. You've done a good job helping your body get well, and what you need to do going forward is to help keep your body in a state in which it can ward off future illness because you don't want to relapse if you can help it. Remember I talked about change? You don't want your body to be in the same circumstances that made you sick in the first place. No, you want to keep transforming your body to where you stack the deck, so to speak, in your favor to put yourself in the best position to avoid illness in the future.

So what do you do now? In short, continue living the lifestyle outlined in this book. Do not let up. Do not take a break. Do not go back to eating and living the way you did before, because if you do, you run the risk of setting yourself up for illness once again. It is better and easier to keep your health than to try to regain it once it is lost. Believe me, I know. You must keep the right mindset—the one in which you will only accept the best for your health. It is this wellness mindset that you must set your mind to in order to set yourself up to walk in super health. I did and you can, too.

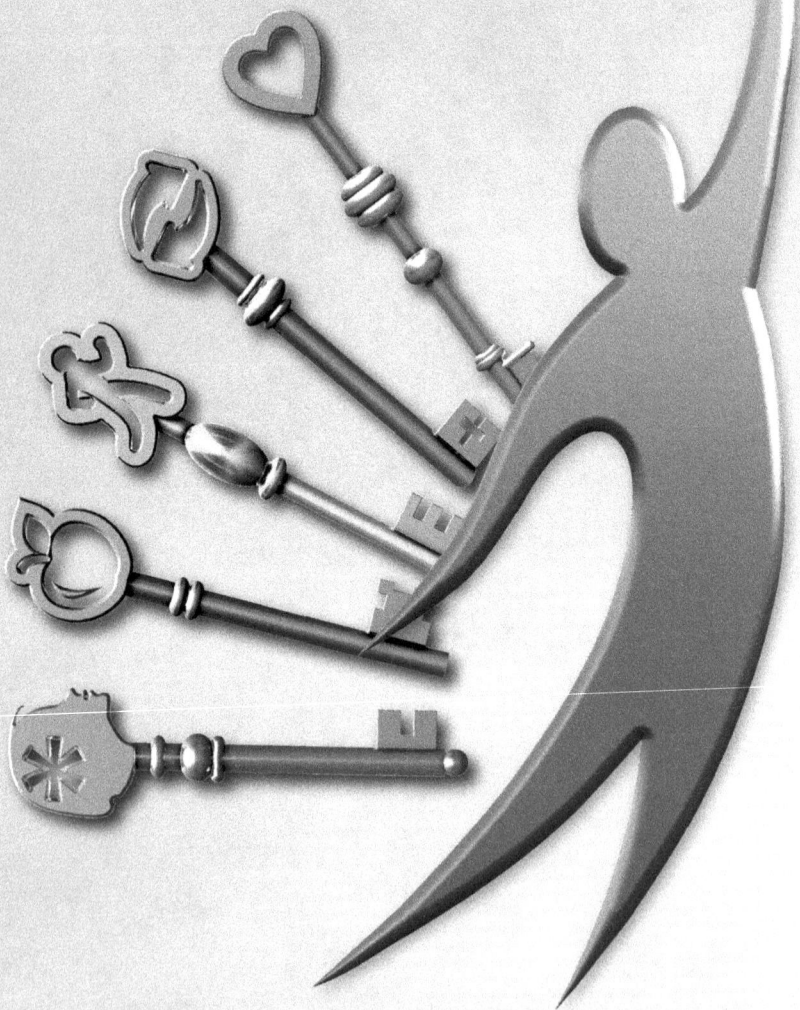

"The ability to find information
and use it wisely to enhance your
health is worth its weight in gold."
— Tracy Kay

RESOURCES

These are some of my favorite resources that I want to share with you.

Recipe Books

I have a great many recipe books, but I turn to these most often:

Eat to Live
Dr. Joel Fuhrman

Vegan Tacos
Jason Wyrick

Forks Over Knives – The Cookbook
Del Sroufe and Isa Chandra Moskowitz

Superfood Kitchen
Julie Morris

The China Study Cookbook
LeAnne Campbell and T. Colin Campbell

The Flavor Bible
Karen Page and Andrew Dornenburg
Note: This isn't a recipe book, but it is an excellent resource for information on how to combine flavors when planning meals.

Whole Food Nutritional Product
One of my doctors put me onto this product during treatment, and it remains a part of my keep-well plan today.
*Juice Plus
Jkay.juiceplus.com

Easy Home Gardening
I grow a ton of fruits and vegetables in a very tiny space using only minerals from the earth and water. No soil needed!
*Tower Garden
Jkay.towergarden.com
I do receive compensation.

VitaMix
www.vitamix.com
You can also find these at www.qvc.com. Many times, QVC will offer the option to pay in installments, which can make this more affordable.

Blendtec
www.blendtec.com

NutriBullet
www.nutribullet.com

Superfoods
www.navitas.com
www.vitacost.com

Learning Resources
Matthew Kenney
Matthew Kenney offers innovative courses on plant-based cuisine at his Santa Monica, CA, location or online.
http://www.matthewkenneycuisine.com

Super Immunity
Dr. Joel Fuhrman
This, in my opinion, should be on everyone's bookshelf. It is especially valuable if you are fighting an illness.

It's Just My Nature
Carol Tuttle
I love this! It's a valuable guide to living true to yourself.

Kitchen Medicine
Julie Bruton-Seal and Matthew Seal
Great information on how everyday foods can enhance your health and beauty.

Personal Care Products
Living Libations
These are amazing and unique personal care products!
www.livinglibations.com

Vitacost
Shopping here, I have found, is in many cases less expensive than buying the same products in health food stores.
www.vitacost.com

Pratima Ayurvedic Skincare
I love these products! I highly recommend the Rose Neem sunscreen.
www.pratimaskincare.com

Some of my favorite products and where to purchase:
Hugo Naturals Fizzy Bath Bombs
Hugo Naturals Dead Sea Salt Scrubs
EO Essential Oil Products Everyone Lotion Unscented
Auromere Herbal Toothpaste
www.vitacost.com

Brad's Kale Chips
Whole Foods

Dr. Fuhrman's G-BOMBS Soups
www.drfuhrman.com

Savvy Rest Organic Bedding
www.savvyrest.com

ACKNOWLEDGMENTS

I knew I had something to say, and I had many voices of encouragement and inspiration behind me as I began to set the words to paper. With this in mind, I want to thank Dr. Sakiliba Mines, MD; Dr. Jay Benson, DO; Dr. Kevin Pett, DOM, Dr. Rosemary Altemus, MD, Dr. David Heyer, MD, and Dr. Henele E'ale, ND, for their expertise and ongoing care when I needed it most. I also want to thank Matthew Kenney for the beauty and knowledge he brings to the world of plant food.

Many thanks to Kira Freed, my incredible editor, for understanding my voice and making my words sing, and to Charlie Alolkoy for bringing my vision to life with his incredible art.

Last and certainly not least, thank you to my family and friends who have been there for me throughout this journey.

www.ingramcontent.com/pod-product-compliance
Lightning Source LLC
Chambersburg PA
CBHW060642280326
41933CB00012B/2116